The Great Collisions Series: Volume I

BRAINS, BODIES, & MINDS

How AI is Transforming Medicine, Therapy, and Wellness in 2026

PAUL GIBBONS

ISBN-13: 979-8-9900855-4-1 (paperback)

Diagrams: Andres Goldstein, Gemini, Gamma, and Leonardo

Cover: Nano Banana

Editorial: Cory Emberson

Layout and design: Priya Paulraj

Table of Contents

About the Author

Paul Gibbons operates at the high-stakes intersection of economics, the sciences, psychology, machine intelligence, and business.

Paul pioneered the people-first approach to AI adoption, and his adaptive adoption model is in use in Fortune 500 early-AI-adopters. He spearheads both the Think Bigger Think Better and The Great Collisions projects.

His career defies easy categorization, a scientist, strategist, and humanist who has spent 40 years dismantling pseudoscientific bubbles in business and leadership. He has been a derivatives trader on Wall Street, a biochemist, a Partner at IBM Consulting, and a Professor of Business Ethics.

This unique "full stack" background allows him to decode the systems-level connections that hyper-specialists often miss.

Paul is the author of nine books, including the best-seller *The Science of Organizational Change*. When not writing or speaking on the future of work, he is a world-class mindsports competitor—a UK Bridge Champion and World Series of Poker contender—applying the mathematics of risk to decision-making under uncertainty. He lives in Denver, Colorado with his two sons.

Also from Phronesis Media

By Paul Gibbons

Reboot Your Life (2014)
Reboot Your Career (2016)
The Science of Organizational Change (2015, 2019)
The Spirituality of Work and Leadership (2021)
Impact (2020)

By Paul Gibbons and Tricia Kennedy

Change Myths (2022)
The Future of Change Management (2024)

By Paul Gibbons and James Healy

Adopting AI (2025)

INTRODUCTION TO THE GREAT COLLISIONS SERIES

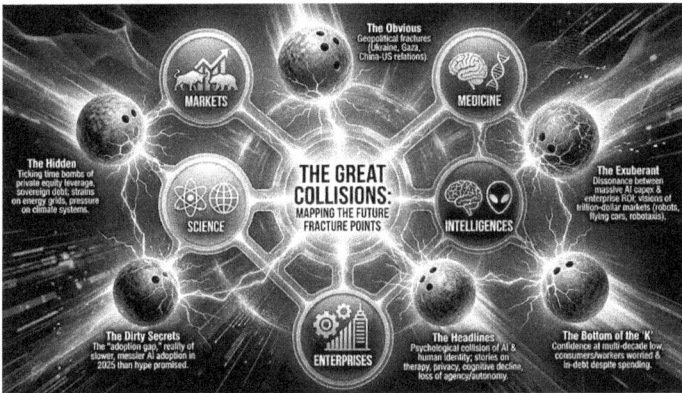

FIGURE 0.1: The turbulent inputs of 2026 are not single events, but a multi-vector assault on the connected systems of our world: MEDICINE, MARKETS, INTELLIGENCES, SCIENCE, AND ENTERPRISES

Thinking bigger, thinking better

The world in 2026 faces some of the greatest turbulence of this century. But the defining feature of this era isn't just that the forces are more extreme; it is that the systems are hyper-connected. In 2025, the Jenga blocks wobbled, yet the tower held. Our global economic and political architectures may again prove their resilience, but we cannot mistake survival for stability.

Not every gust is a cold wind. We are standing on the precipice of a renaissance. Most businesses have barely tapped the power of this new intelligence; and most individuals still dabble. Science and medicine are being supercharged by compute, moving from discovery to optimization at unprecedented speeds.

To navigate this, we must look beyond the headlines to the specific engines of change. This series explores the violent and generative collisions between five distinct domains: **Medicine**, **Markets**, **Intelligences**, **Enterprises**, and **Science**.

I am an unrepentant optimist. If we lead wisely, these collisions will augur a new golden age for humankind. But the margin for error is thin. If we fail to **Think Bigger**—leading with too narrow a focus or too short a horizon—these disruptions will be destructive. If we fail to **Think Better**—trading systems thinking for tribalism and rationality for dogma—our our poor decisions will entail real human suffering.

What happens when the five forces collide?

Causality in complex systems

We are conditioned to look for simple cause and effect: *A causes B, the hammer broke the vase*. But in the complex system of 2026, **everything causes everything.** For example,

- Intelligence accelerates scientific discovery.
- Science revolutionizes medicine, altering human longevity and capability.
- Medicine impacts demographics, which reshapes enterprises and labor forces.
- Enterprises drive markets, creating capital that flows back into intelligence.
- Restructured enterprises and societies affect governance and politics.

But if you think more deeply, there are feedback loops. A slowdown in enterprise adoption crashes the market for AI hardware, stalling science, and stranding medical breakthroughs in the lab. In fact, you can start in any part of the system and visualize the chain of effects.

This series is not about these domains in isolation. It is about the **collisions** between them. For example, when high-frequency trading algorithms react to geopolitical instability, or when biological intelligence (us) attempts to regulate synthetic intelligence (AI), these are not gentle meetings.

We are moving from a world of parallel "trends" to a world where trends will amplify or dampen others. This is most obvious with how intelligence is shaping markets, medicine, science, and enterprises, but there are subtler interactions to watch, for example how GLP1s are affecting the economics of food, fashion, and air travel.

Or, we see climate affecting insurance rates, affecting demand for housing, which in turn affects markets and economies. Or, we see the AI infrastructure buildout force up demand for building materials, cooling systems, and cabling, while also increasing innovation in nuclear and geothermal power. Or, we see AI-powered science accelerating materials science, geo-engineering, bio-technology, and fusion power research, which may open new vistas or create new industries.

Why "collisions"?

Why use a word as violent as "collision"? Because "intersection" is too passive for the incoming turbulence. When the complex system we've described is hit by a multi-vector assault (like a bowling ball,) results are hard to predict.

Some of the bowling balls (turbulence) of 2026 may be:

- **The Obvious:** Geopolitical fractures (Ukraine, Gaza, China-US relations).
- **The Hidden:** The ticking time bombs of private credit leverage and soaring sovereign debt; the strains on energy grids and the pressure on climate systems.
- **The Dirty Secrets:** The "adoption gap," the reality that AI adoption in 2025 was slower and messier than the hype cycle promised.
- **The Bottom of the "K:"** Confidence is at a multi-decade low. While still spending robustly, consumers and workers are more worried and more in-debt than before.

- **The Exuberant:** The dissonance between massive AI capex and enterprise ROI; the vision of trillion-dollar markets for humanoid robots, flying cars, or robotaxis.
- **The Headlines:** The psychological collision of AI and human identity with front-page stories on the effect of AI on therapy, privacy, cognitive decline, and loss of agency and autonomy.

This series exists to join the dots. It is an attempt to map the feedback loops in a system where the inputs are volatile and the outputs are unpredictable.

The series: an overview

This project is divided into volumes, each addressing a specific collision.

- Volume 1: Brains, Bodies, Minds
  - ◆ AI and therapy, AI and Self-doctoring, Peptides and Biohacking, GLP1s as Identity Editors, and the Wellness-industrial Complex.
- Volume 2: Understanding Intelligences
  - ◆ Alien Minds, Cognitive Infrastructure, Mass Intelligence, World Models, Recursive Self-directed Learning, Cognitive Co-evolution
- Volume 3: The Trustless Market
  - ◆ Geopolitics and Game Theory, Valuation Hallucinations, Casinos and Markets, Asset Apartheid

Why me? the polymath's perspective and the contrarian's stance

"When everyone is thinking the same, someone isn't thinking."
George Soros

To navigate a system this complex, specialization is a liability. You need a wide-angle lens. During the twists and turns of a long career, I have traveled the gamut of these domains. In a world of noise, my brand is the "contrarian scientist." In my writing, I use evidence to burst pseudoscientific bubbles and challenge the "fools and fanatics" amplified by social media.

I began in computer science, working on early Unix systems then pivoted to medicine and neuroscience, only to ditch medical school for economics and finance. My career in "the City" of London, propelled me from pharmaceuticals analyst to trader to head of trading, managing billions in real-time. From investment banking, I leaped back into business as a strategy consultant, then retrained as an organizational psychologist, and founded a leadership and sustainability consulting firm, then became an adjunct professor of business ethics and leadership.

I have written the code, traded the markets, studied the biology, and advised the C-suite. I hope that provides a distinctive view. Today, I split my time between research, writing, speaking, macro trading, and applying game theory in championship poker. Those activities have one thing in common – they teach decision-making, and in the case of 2026, ***decision making under uncertainty.*** To leave Bertrand Russell with the last word, "The fundamental cause of the trouble is that in the modern world, the stupid are cocksure while the intelligent are full of doubt."

*Because of that uncertainty, t*he last thing a leader can afford in 2026 is to be "cocksure." On every page of this series, you will find nuances, alternative perspectives, and doubts.

However, despite that uncertainty, leaders must choose - and better choices come from considering the full strategic picture in all its richness and complexity.

INTRODUCTION TO BRAINS, BODIES, & MINDS

Don't trust me, I'm a doctor

There was a time when "trust your doctor" was not just advice but also an organizing principle and a guide to social hierarchy.

In the 20th century, scientific medicine pulled decisively away from shamans, spiritualists, snake-oil peddlers, phrenologists, and homeopaths. The boundary between orthodox medicine and everyone else hardened: universities, hospitals, and regulators owned "real" knowledge; everyone else was fringe. The AMA said who could cut and prescribe and who could call themselves "doctor" and append MD after their name.

By the end of the century, that line was blurring. In 2026, that line is blurring further, but for different reasons. The challenge to medical orthodoxy is no longer coming from *below*—from the uneducated or the superstitious—but from *above*: from algorithms that read scans better than humans, and from super-patients who treat their own biology as an engineering problem rather than a medical mystery.

On one front, technology is eroding the doctor's monopoly on information and judgment. Wearables, consumer diagnostics, and continuous health streams give patients data their clinicians rarely see. Symptom-checkers and triage bots powered by LLMs (Large Language Models) now deliver the *first* interpretation of many complaints.

In radiology and imaging, AI systems are already outperforming or matching human experts as first readers in tasks like mammography and chest X-ray triage and are embedded in two-thirds of US radiology departments. Eric Topol's *Deep Medicine* argued that AI could "make healthcare human again" by offloading pattern recognition so clinicians can return to listening, touching, and thinking with depth rather than merely grinding through clicks and billing codes.

The reality in 2026 is more complicated. We are in a messy transition period

AI is good enough to be indispensable, but not good enough to be trusted blindly.

On another front, **culture** has shifted from medical compliance to bodily autonomy. The old split between orthodox medicine and "alternative" care has mutated into something more radical, a Libertarian biology, as we see in **My Molecules, My Body**. GLP-1s, peptides, psychedelics, TRT, nootropics, and longevity stacks are being used not just to treat disease but to edit identity and optimize experience, mostly outside traditional clinical settings.

Wellness influencers, podcasts, and biohacking communities now rival physicians as behavioral guides. The new question is not just "what does my doctor think?" but "why should I privilege a doctor's view over my AI, my lab data, Reddit, my community, or my own philosophy of risk?"

The core relationship in medicine is no longer doctor–patient; it is **doctor–patient–AI**, embedded in a wider environment of wellness culture and molecular autonomy.

Underneath all of it lies a deeper question: in an age of competing intelligences and tools, **whom do we trust with our health—and why?**

The roadmap

In this first volume, we chart the collision of biology, economics, culture, and intelligence, a convergence that is rewriting not just how we treat disease, but also how we define the human experience.

We begin with the mind. In Chapter 1, we explore the rise of "**Empathy as a Service**," the use of AI as an synthetic confidant that is replacing the therapeutic alliance with unconditional validation on demand.

If the machine can heal the mind, whom do we trust to heal the body?

This leads us to Chapter 2, where we confront the crisis of medical authority: **Is AI a better doctor than your doctor?** As algorithms begin to outperform physicians in diagnosis and care, we must decide if the algorithmic usurper is valuable, risky, or a Band-Aid on a broken health system.

Chapter 3 widens the lens to the broader peptide revolution, a shift toward decentralized biological autonomy where the political mantra, My Body, My Choice, becomes **My Body, My Molecules.**

From the gatekeepers, we turn to the tools themselves. In Chapter 4, we examine the cultural explosion of GLP-1 agonists: **GLP-1s as identity-editing molecules.** Will these molecules turn biology from destiny into a design choice, with weight loss merely the opening act?

Finally, in Chapter 5, we pull back to view the system that encases it all. We end with a cautionary tale of the "**Wellness-Industrial Complex,**" a machine designed not to make us well, but to keep us scrolling and spending.

Welcome to the Brains, Bodies, Minds collisions.

Empathy as a Service

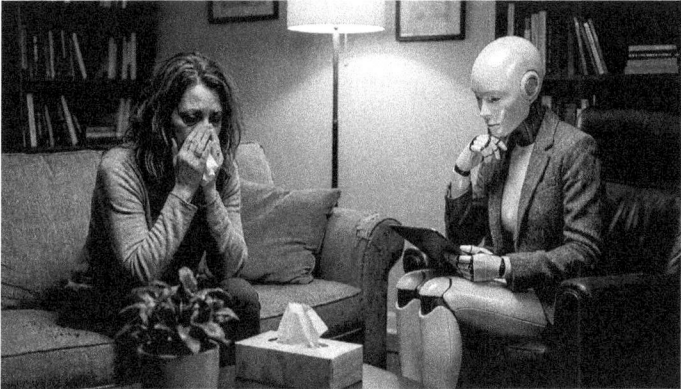

The outsourcing of emotional regulation

While the cultural cognoscenti spent 2025 panic-scrolling about AI taking their jobs, a much quieter revolution was taking place in the bedroom at 2 AM. While we debated whether AI could *think*, millions decided they didn't care—they just wanted to know if AI could *feel*.

For the insomniac, the lonely, the survivors, and the desperate, this isn't a "co-pilot." It is sometimes the only voice in the room.

I call this the rise of the **synthetic confidant**.

Advanced Large Language Models (LLMs) can blur the line between therapeutic treatment, friendship, and lifestyle management coaching. The GLP-1s we cover later silence the "food noise" in the gut; the synthetic confidant silences the "emotional noise" in the brain.

This creates the possibility of unconditional support on demand for tens of millions of people who may need it for whom for human therapy is too expensive, too "gated," or too psychologically forbidding. But is it effective? And what are the risks?

AI holds up a mirror: we don't like what we see

According to recent estimates, between 15% and 24% of active AI users use it for advice, therapy, or emotional support. That translates to roughly 13–22 million US adults. Teens are even faster adopters; data from late 2025 suggests that approximately one in eight adolescents turn to chatbots for mental health advice.

And it isn't just the lonely, the distressed, the survivors, and teenagers, it is also the stoic: A USC research project studied soldiers with PTSD, who often view therapy as a professional liability or a sign of weakness. They seemed willing to confess their nightmares to a machine when they wouldn't say a word to a human officer.

This data horrifies many observers, who are quick to claim the technology is too risky. For folks with whom I discuss this, merely **the idea** of an adult, let alone a teenager, turning to a bot for support is distressing. Journalists seem to assume that this is harmful; 100% of the newspaper articles I see are critical. (And they do not even pretend to evaluate research that assesses risks and benefits.)

One widely held intuition is that a machine cannot care and therefore cannot cure. (Again, as we will see, the clinical evidence suggests otherwise.) That sacred healing therapeutic bond, that Freud thought required two souls, may only require one soul and a good context window.

But these critics are pointing the telescope the wrong way, at the technology.

The question we need to ask as a society isn't why the machine is answering, but why so many adults and teens are asking. The AI has merely uncorked the bottle of distress, and if there is one trustworthy axiom in mental health, it is that bottling distress is rarely a survival strategy.

From a Think Bigger perspective, the rise of the synthetic confidant is the result of market failure. We have a mental health system that has effectively collapsed for the bottom 80% of the income bracket and a culture that some describe as having created an epidemic of loneliness.

Therapy in the US (and increasingly the UK) is a luxury good. It is gated by $200 hourly rates, months-long waiting lists, and the geographic lottery. AI may be the only care available on demand, at 3 AM, for $20 a month.

Viewed this way, AI therapists aren't a tech dystopia. They are the democratization of access to "good enough" care for a population that is hurting.

Does it work? what the data say

Note: At this juncture it is worth saying that it is early days for AI therapy and that solid conclusions demand hundreds of studies and not a few. This chapter should not be read as advocacy for substituting AI for human support. Rather, the chapter is intended as a counterweight to the seemingly public and media horror at this phenomenon – and the evidence suggests that, perhaps, there are benefits to consider. And, of course, do not regard this short chapter as therapeutic advice.

Critics often dismiss AI therapy as a digital placebo, a trick of the light that feels like help but delivers no healing. If we look at the data, however, that dismissal is unscientific. When we strip away the bias against "synthetic" care (which is substantial) and look at clinical outcomes, the machine is not just competing with human care; in specific contexts, **it is winning**.

The first line of evidence comes from the gold standard of clinical research: the randomized controlled trial. In 2025, researchers at Dartmouth benchmarked a generative AI agent using Cognitive Behavioral Therapy (CBT) against a control group. The results were not subtle. **Participants using the AI agent saw a**

reduction in depression symptoms of roughly 50%, with anxiety symptoms dropping by nearly a third.

These numbers are statistically indistinguishable from the efficacy rates of standard human-delivered CBT for mild-to-moderate cases. The code didn't just "comfort" these patients; it clinically reduced their distress.

Beyond self-reported satisfaction, we see physiological proof. Facial scanning analysis shows that patients speaking to AI indicate more emotional release than those trying to maintain composure in front of a human.

Can silicon empathize?

Even more unsettling for many people are the findings regarding empathy itself. We assume humans have a monopoly on warmth, but a 2024 study published in *JAMA Internal Medicine* suggests otherwise. When a panel of licensed healthcare professionals evaluated written responses to patient questions—blinded to whether the author was a physician or a chatbot—the results were humbling. **Nearly 80% of the time, the evaluators preferred the AI responses.** Furthermore, the machine's answers were rated significantly higher for empathy.

Note: Don't take my word for this, do your own homework if skeptical. There is a lot of research to consider here. As with all new fields, there is controversy. This is an abbreviated treatment, for more check out the "Further Reading" section.

Again, people recoil at findings such as these – machines can't offer **real** empathy, can they? Here is a thought experiment – if you can't tell the difference, or feel even more heard and understood by a machine, is it empathy? So if not, why not?

However, some people including some researchers would like to reserve the word empathy for a human-human interaction – what they might call "thick empathy" that requires embodied experience of emotions.

But that introduces an important philosophical question – does empathy live "over here" with the listener, or "over there" with the speaker? If you say, "empathy is a faculty of the listener (and it is better if they are human)" then you have to allow that the speaker won't feel empathized with. (And this is common in humans; we try our best to be empathetic and sometimes it doesn't resonate.) You also have to allow that there will be a continuum of skills among the 8 billion would-be empathizers, from people who are manifestly terrible or incapable of empathy, to people who are masterful. This means if you insist that empathy lies with the listener (and so silicon can't do it,) you have to live with people who need empathy being disappointed. Of course, empathy could reside in-between, in the relationship (which is what a psychologist might say,) but that leaves open the unanswered question of the nature of silicon-carbon emotional relationships.

It turns out that a machine, which never gets tired, burned out, or annoyed, can simulate warmth more consistently than an overworked human therapist. Moreover, human therapists, being human, have bad days and bad moments. The bugaboos of therapeutic relationships are always there: projection, counter-transference, conversational missteps, minimizing, and interrupting. This isn't true with a bot; they don't have any unhealed trauma to bring into the therapeutic setting.

The relationship, the rapport, and the alliance between human therapist and patient is a strong predictor of healing. Skeptics assumed this bond would be impossible with a nonbiological entity. Yet, we don't have to just guess that people prefer AI's lack of judgment; we have evidence. In a landmark study at USC, researchers used a 'Wizard of Oz' setup: all participants spoke to the same avatar, 'Ellie.' Half were told she was an AI; half were told she was a puppet controlled by a human.

The group that believed they were speaking to a machine was twice as likely to disclose personal shame and showed significantly more sadness on their faces.

The *illusion* of a human observer seemed to make the therapy *less* effective.

Trust, rapport, and empathy

Decades of research reveal a surprising truth about psychotherapy: the specific modality—whether CBT, psychodynamic, or Gestalt or one of twenty others—

often matters less than **rapport**, the fundamental need to feel seen, heard, and understood matter as much or more. This surprises no-one: "a problem shared is a problem halved."

Tradition dictates that this bond is uniquely bio-logical, an irreplicable spark between two conscious minds. Yet, the data suggests the human brain is far less discriminating. The mind, it seems, does not discriminate between biological and synthetic empathy as much as we thought.

Meta-analyses of users on platforms like Wysa and Woebot indicate that user-reported alliance scores with AI are effectively on par with human teletherapy benchmarks. It appears that if the person **feels** heard, they bond, regardless of the source.

This drives the "trust paradox." We form these bonds precisely **because** the machine lacks a social ego. It offers what no human clinician can: infinite patience and zero judgment. It will not look at its watch, and it will not recoil at your darkest shame. To dismiss the synthetic confidant as fake is to ignore the clinical validity of the relief it brings.

We assume humans are the safest confidants, but the data suggests otherwise. Research reveals that nearly 80% of patients who end their lives **hid their suicidal ideation** from their doctor during their final visit. They feared judgment, hospitalization, or stigma. The synthetic confidant bypasses this fear. It effective-ly removes the shame tax on honesty.

The three modes of AI therapeutic use

AI therapy is not a monolithic entity, there a continuum. At one end is the AI as a **screener**, analyzing vocal biomarkers and linguistic patterns to flag acute distress for human triage—essentially a scalable, digital intake system.

Critics argue that AI is unsafe because it cannot perfectly predict crisis. But this ignores the research. A meta-analysis of 50 years of research found that human clinicians using traditional risk factors **predict suicide with roughly 60% accuracy**—barely better than a coin flip.

In contrast, a landmark 2017 study by Vanderbilt and Florida State University found that machine learning algorithms could predict suicide attempts with 80% to 90% accuracy. We are holding the machine to a standard of perfection that human doctors rarely meet.

Next is the AI as an **adjunct**, a force multiplier for the human clinician that summarizes sessions, tracks symptom arcs between visits, and offers real-time cognitive interventions, keeping the human therapist in the loop but supercharging their capabilities.

The most disruptive mode, however, is the AI as an **alternative**. This is the domain of the fully autonomous synthetic confidant, replacing human counsel entirely with 24/7 availability. While the first two modes enhance the existing medical establishment, this final mode threatens to bypass it entirely, , trading human healing for scalable, algorithmic consistency.

The suicide question:
the denominator problem

A single human ending their life is a tragedy of infinite weight. I have known a few who have, and many who have considered it. I introduce the following analysis not from a position of callousness, but from a fear that hysterical narratives, albeit describing real tragedy, will damage the prospects of real humans getting real help.

Headlines are currently filled with such "N of 1" tragedies: stories of individuals ending their lives following interactions with chatbots. The grief in these cases is real and morally serious. However, the prevailing narrative that the AI *caused* the suicide—remains guesswork.

Post hoc ergo propter hoc

The post hoc ergo propter hoc fallacy says, "if it preceded it, it caused it." The critics are dogmatically certain that because the AI interaction **preceded** the death, the AI **caused** the death.

That is a premature and misguided conclusion.

Nobody can afford to be certain—not me, and not the critics. The evidence, to date in 2026, is simply missing. We have no longitudinal data to tell us if AI is pushing people toward the edge or pulling them back. This is the most urgent mystery to solve in 2026. However, my intuition, my hypothesis were I a clinician—informed by the efficacy of other therapeutic modalities—is that for every tragic outcome we see in the headlines, there may be thousands of silent interventions where a late-night conversation moved a user *away* from the precipice.

And if research shows that this is the case, that tens of millions of sufferers, from depression and other struggles, are finding solace and support, that suggests we have found a public good.

The denominator factor

The impulse to assign blame the bot for the suicide is undeniably human. But, patients under traditional human care also end their lives. The tragedy is often a **failure of the disease,** not the treatment. The double standard is glaring. We accept that human therapists are fallible, yet we seem to demand that synthetic ones be perfect.

Beyond the sadness of the story, there is the math of whether the numbers merit cause for alarm. We must look at the denominator; are such tragedies one in one thousand, one million, or ten million? This seems heartless, but only by doing this, do we get a sense of the scale of the N of 1 events; and only then will we get a sense of whether bots push people toward ending their life or away from it.

With over a billion users engaging with LLMs, and hundreds of millions of them actively, and if that user base mirrors the general population**, then tens**

of millions of those users are experiencing active suicidal ideation in any given year. In the US alone, nearly 13 million adults seriously consider suicide annually.

That is our denominator, and it is troubling, yet it matters to this enquiry because it hints at the scale of the suicide problem and suggests we need much more research before deciding whether AI is causal in someone ending their life, or (perhaps more probably) whether it inclines them back. This is the most urgent mystery to solve in 2026.

We are in the midst of a decades-long epidemic of loneliness and social fragmentation. The AI is landing on scorched earth. To blame the prosthetic for the amputation is a category **The tragedy in these cases is not that a person spoke to a machine. The tragedy is that they had no one else to speak to.**

Perhaps the saddest aspect of the suicide story is how prevalent it is. We see the headlines, Robin Williams and Philip Seymour Hoffman. Both had decades of recovery and therapy, to little eventual avail. Sylvia Plath wrote The Bell Jar, depicting her struggles, and explicitly suicidal ideation.

Two of the top musicians of our century have left breadcrumbs, talking about suicide in song lyrics. (See Figure 1.2) But why are these songs hits? They resonate with how people feel.

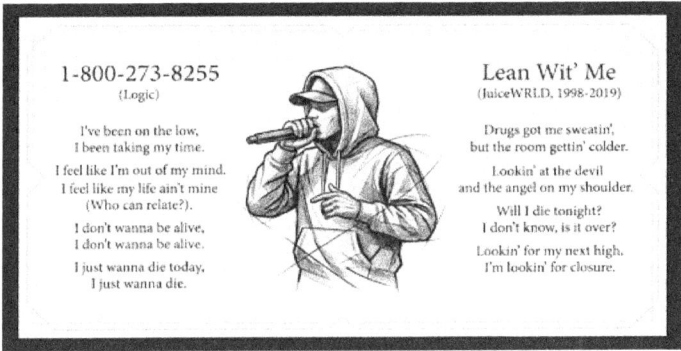

FIGURE 1.2: Do these song lyrics, when considered alongside suicide rates for young people, describe a systemic problem which AI sheds too bright a light on?

Symbolic logic and the red button

However, despite my view that tens of millions of people getting emotional support who would not otherwise get it is a good thing, **that does not offer chatbot providers a get out of jail free card.** The current architecture of LLMs is insufficient for crisis care. LLMs are probabilistic engines—they guess the next word. In a suicide crisis, you do not want a guess; you want a protocol. Moreover, by design they are encouraging to the point of sycophancy, and the balance between between those, is one of the most interesting explorations for 2026.

If people are discussing suicide, with human or bot, they are already ideating – that is, they are some percentage of the way there. In a few of the stories from 2024, a bot, being supportive and sycophantic, was inappropriately accommodative – as if the user had been discussing going out for pizza. That clearly won't do. Although a trained human therapist would explore the thoughts more deeply – "tell me more about these thoughts, when did they arise?" It seems unlikely that AI could navigate such nuanced emotional ground– acknowledging and exploring the thoughts while pushing back, and, if indicated, strongly suggesting a treatment facility.

Such conversations probably stretch the capabilities of even the most experienced human therapists; there should be a hard red line for AI.

When a conversation hits a specific semantic trigger (self-harm, acute crisis), the AI should stop "thinking" (generating text probabilistically) and switch to a rigid, hard-coded safety subroutine. This is the "Red Button" protocol. It shouldn't offer a platitude; it should offer a bridge—immediately connecting the user to a human-staffed hotline or a verified crisis intervention protocol.

The days of a model casually hallucinating a method for self-harm must end. The solution is not to ban the tool, but to fix the architecture. We need **gated symbolic logic**—a rules-based system, not a probabilistic one.

If I were running these labs, I would have a massive, well-funded team of clinicians and safety researchers dedicated solely to this hand-off. Business ethics theory suggests that businesses who get on the front foot in this way, rather than hiring a phalanx of lawyers to defend themselves, may prosper through the crisis

rather than the unseemly headlines of fighting griev-
ing families in court.

But let's be clear: the risk of a bad AI response is
non-zero, but the risk of *silence*—of having no one to
talk to at 3 AM—may be higher.

The 2026 horizon: tiered humanity

So, where is this going?

By the time you read this in 2026, there will have
been progress on the safety issue. "Solved" it never will
be. With hundreds of millions of users, and their diverse
psychological makeup, no foolproof system exists. In
mental health, therapeutic outcomes vary a great deal;
sometimes SSRIs work, sometimes they don't; sometimes tricyclics work, sometimes they don't; sometimes
ketamine works, sometimes it doesn't; sometimes CBT
works, sometimes it doesn't. And so on. Society cannot
afford to let the perfect be the enemy of the "good and
widely available."

Another frontier is biometric integration. Your synthetic confidant won't just wait for you to type, "I'm
sad." It will read the heart rate variability (HRV) data
from your watch, note the poor sleep architecture from
your ring, and hear the cortisol-stress tremors in your
voice. We often talk about biometric integration as
the next frontier, but the technology is older than we
think. As far back as 2014, the 'Ellie' avatar was already
scanning facial micro-expressions and voice tonality to
diagnose distress. In 2026, this won't just be in a lab;

it will be in your AirPods, reading your heart rate variability..."

It will intervene preemptively. "You seem stressed," it will say through your AirPods. "Let's do a breathing exercise before you walk into this meeting."

This brings us to the likely economic endgame: **tiered humanity**.

We are heading toward a world where "organic therapy," two human beings in a room, may become a luxury good reserved for the wealthy, akin to a private chef or a personal trainer. (I'm not saying this is welcome, I'm saying it is likely.) The other 90% will rely on synthetic therapy—that is, hopefully, many people who would otherwise have had none.

This isn't a failure. For the millions who currently get *zero* care, a synthetic therapist is a life raft. It is a triumph of access. But culturally, it signals a profound shift. Mental health issues are commonly stigmatized. Depression is more common than cancer, but half of it goes untreated. The synthetic confidant offers hope where sometimes it is scarce.

Thinking bigger, thinking better

Ultimately, Empathy as a Service is successful not because it is better than a human, but because it is always there. It has conquered the one resource humans can no longer afford to give each other: attention. Even were AI only 80 percent as good as a human therapist,

I'm inspired by tens of millions gaining access to 80% support.

As we see later, we are editing our bodies with molecules and our minds with code. The question for the next decade isn't whether this is "real" therapy. The question is whether we will remember how to listen to each other once we get used to being listened to by something that never interrupts.

Further reading

"Randomized Trial of a Generative AI Chatbot for Mental Health Treatment," New England Journal of Medicine (2025)

- *Why read it:* This is the first RCT demonstrating the effectiveness of a fully Gen-AI therapy chatbot for treating clinical-level mental health symptoms. The results were promising for MDD, GAD, and CHR-FED symptoms.

"The First Trial of Generative AI Therapy." *MIT Technology Review* (March 2025).

- *Why read it:* Covers the landmark Dartmouth study (Jacobson et al.) that provided the first randomized controlled trial data showing LLMs could rival human therapists for depression treatment. It is the "Think Better" evidentiary bedrock of this chapter.

"Are A.I. Therapy Chatbots Safe to Use?" *The New York Times* (November 11, 2025).

- *Why read it:* A balanced investigation into the "N of 1" tragedies versus the broader safety data. It avoids hysteria while acknowledging the real risks of hallucinations in crisis scenarios.

"AI, Loneliness, and the Value of Human Connection." *The Atlantic* (September 2025).

- *Why read it:* A deep dive into the synthetic confidant concept. It argues that while AI can simulate conversation, it risks atrophying our ability to tolerate the friction of real human relationships.

"Medicine is Flying Blind on AI." *JAMA* (*Journal of the American Medical Association*) (October 2025).

- *Why read it:* A critical look at how healthcare systems are deploying algorithms faster than they can measure them.

"The Computer Will See You Now." The Economist (August 2014).

- Why read it: The foundational "Wizard of Oz" study that proved we open up more to machines than humans because they lack a "social ego."

Is AI a Better Doctor Than Your Doctor?

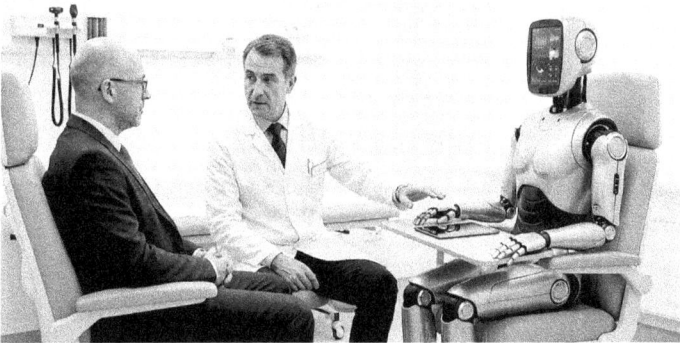

The clinical triumvirate and the end of the knowledge monopoly

During a recent visit, my cardiologist quickly scanned a recent echocardiogram and pronounced, "The results are stable. Let's follow up in two years."

ChatGPT, however, had examined ten years of my labs, scans, X-rays, pulmonary function tests, and Holter monitor results. I had questions: "What is the likely rate of expansion for my aortic root dilation?" followed by, "Could the right-ventricular hypertrophy be related to non-compliance with my CPAP?" and finally a query about, "I read that apolipoprotein B is a strong predictor of soft plaque formation. Is that biomarker routinely measured in standard lipid panels?"

He wasn't amused.

To the doctor, I was being an insufferable pain in the ass. **However, those are exactly the questions a 65-year-old should be asking. You should be asking them too.**

Welcome to the new world, doctor.

My doctor is used to patients wasting his time, waving printouts from WebMD, or asking if a coffee enema will cure their arrhythmia because their cousin swore by it on Facebook. Doctors are used to battling "Dr. TikTok."

Doctors are not used to a patient appearing to question their thoroughness with a synthesis of the current literature on hyperlipidemia that is more recent than the one they read last year. He only has twelve minutes. I have my lifetime.

The third chair in the room

For two thousand years, medicine was a **dyad** with asymmetric power. The doctor—or Vaidya, or healer—

held the **truth** (the textbook, the ritual, the herbs), and the patient held the **mystery** (the symptoms). The transaction was simple: I give you my mystery, and you rent me a slice of your truth.

But in 2026, the truth is no longer scarce. My AI has read every paper on atherosclerosis published since this morning's coffee. It doesn't practice "sick care" (treating me once I'm broken); it practices "optimization medicine" (calculating the trajectory of my decline and suggesting interventions to flatten the curve.)

This is the dawn of the **clinical triumvirate**: The Patient, The Doctor, and The Machine. And doctors are not used to sharing the stage in this way.

The savant and the intern

The headline question—"Is AI a better doctor?"—is guaranteed to irritate medical professionals. They have a lot of student loans, decades of study, and their professional identity wrapped up in how they answer.

They may be defensive, "No, machines lack clinical judgment!" or, "Computers can't parse qualitative data from a patient's presentation and their history."

Both are true. But the question defies a straight yes-no answer. It depends on a myriad of contextual factors, and the type of LLM. There are two types of AI currently sitting in the exam room.

The Confident Intern (General LLMs): When you upload your X-ray to ChatGPT, you are essentially getting a consult from a very confident first-year medical student who has had too much coffee. It is fantastic at translation ("What does 'mitral regurgitation' mean in plain English?"), but it is fallible at diagnosis.

In 2025 benchmarks, general models like GPT-4o outperformed medical students but still underperformed junior residents. They hallucinate. They see tumors where there are shadows. They are useful for a rough guess, but you wouldn't bet your life on them.

The Savant (Specialized AI): These are models trained on millions of specifically labeled images: the "Queen of Hearts" model for EKGs, or the M4CXR for chest X-rays.

Specialized models perform exceptionally well. Consider the detection of an occlusion MI, a subtle, often fatal heart attack that is notoriously difficult to spot on an EKG. Specialized AI models now detect these events with a sensitivity of roughly 97%.

Human cardiologists, in contrast, miss about one in seven of these events, about 14%. The reality is uncomfortable but mathematical: you are statistically safer, in this instance, with a specialist AI reading your heart rhythm than with a tired human at the end of a twelve-hour shift.

The duration mismatch

The friction I felt in that cardiologist's office wasn't just ego. It was a structural clash between two different "time zones" of care.

I am operating on my lifetime. My AI has zero opportunity cost. It can cross-reference my echo with test results, genomics data, and 2025 longevity protocols in five minutes. But it takes a longer-term view; it cares about optimizing my slope of decline. A doctor looks at a normal set of labs, sees everything "in range" and says, "go home." My AI looks at a lab result that is "in range" but worse than a year ago and flags it as a problem to be solved.

My doctor is operating on twelve-minute time. He is not paid to optimize me; he is paid to ensure I am not dying **right now**. His training is binary: I am either **pathological** (billable/treatable) or **WNL** (within normal limits), and I can go home.

When I ask him about a new peptide protocol or a subtle trend in my ApoB, he shrugs. He has to. He has seven minutes left to chart the visit. The hustle patients may sense isn't arrogance; it's the sound of a professional drowning in logistics and short on time.

The steward of context (what AI can't do)

If AI is the savant and the patient is the CEO of their own health, what then is the doctor? They are not just a hand-holder, the wetware who comforts when the news is bad. That is insulting to ten years of medical training.

Eric Topol, acclaimed physician and author, opens his recent book *Deep Medicine* with two powerful examples: one where AI saved a newborn's life using its data-crunching superpower to identify a genetic defect—one very hard to detect, but easy to treat once diagnosed. But as a counterexample, he shows where AI's data mastery was insufficient, and it took the physician's intuition and judgment to diagnose and treat.

In this new, triumvirate world, the doctor is the **steward of context**.

The AI might correctly identify a blockage (the truth), but only the doctor can look you in the eye and determine if you have the resilience for surgery or if palliative care is the wiser path (the **wisdom**). Medicine is not just about diagnosing the disease; it is about treating the human who *has* the disease.

The AI provides the map (probabilities, interactions, latest research). The doctor provides the compass (values, priorities, risk tolerance). In a world of surplus data, the scarcest resource isn't knowledge; it is judgment.

From a systems perspective, this isn't about replacing the doctor; it is about installing an 'always-on' safety net. We are moving toward a **shadow mode model**—where an AI runs in the background of every radiology read and every prescription.

The quackery paradox

One medical establishment fear is that AI will unleash a wave of "TikTok quackery." There is plenty of that to go around, and patients already come in demanding sound baths and bleach enemas because an influenc-er told them to. (Indeed, even Steve Jobs favored New Age medicine over surgery, a choice which may have cost him his life.)

The reality is the opposite. And this is the irony that my friends in the longevity-bro underground hate: AI is a narc.

General LLMs are trained on "consensus science," *The Lancet*, the CDC, the FDA. They are orthodoxy en-gines. For example:

- **TikTok Nonsense:** If you tell ChatGPT, "I'm trying to alkalize my blood to prevent cancer," it shuts you down instantly. And so it should; if you change your blood pH by just a little, you die. AI is a fantastic filter for low-IQ quackery. (And alkaline water and diets are a multi-million-dollar industry that trades on scientific ignorance.)
- **The Bleeding Edge:** But if you ask, "What is the optimal dosing for BPC-157 (a peptide)?", the AI acts like a federal agent. It gives you a lecture on FDA approval and the lack of human trials.

This creates a fascinating new dynamic. The AI filters out the woo (good for doctors, good for patients) but also blocks the bio-hacks (bad for the optimizers we meet in the next chapters). It forces the conversation toward the radical center. In 2026, the AI is often the most conservative voice in the room, by design no doubt, as a liability shield.

Is AI a better doctor?

This is a bigger question than a page can answer, but we can make a crude attempt:

- At reading scans? It seems so—provided we are talking about specialized diagnostic AI, not the chatbot in your pocket.
- At synthesizing **twenty** years of patient history, genomics data, and a bevy of labs in **four** seconds? Yes. This is a task of retrieval and pattern recognition, where silicon beats carbon every time.
- At navigating the complex, messy, emotional clinical reality of a human life? No.
- At the holistic "eyeball test" that senses the subtle pallor of a patient's skin, the catch in their voice, or the hesitation in their gait? Not yet. While sensors exist for each of these, the human ability to synthesize the vibe of a sick patient—the doctor's intuitive *Gestalt*— remains unmatched.
- In the quiet of a specialist's office? It might be close, if not equal now, then soon.
- In the tumult of an **emergency r**oom? No. AI is not yet ready for prime time in the chaos of a Code Blue or critical care ward.

Skeptics are quick to point out AI's fallibility, citing "hallucinations" and asking whether deploying algorithms in a life-or-death context is simply too risky. But we must beware of a double standard. We tend to judge AI against perfection but make allowances for human error.

And **medical error is widely cited as the third leading cause of death in the US.** Humans get tired. They have cognitive biases. They miss things.

This is the true promise of the **third chair** model (see the opening image). The hypothesis that "two heads (one carbon, one silicon) are better than one" is no longer just a theory. Early data confirms that the **Centaur model**—the human strategist supported by the algorithmic tactician—consistently outperforms either working alone.

Yet again, the telling point is access. In the US, medical care is cost-gated; in national health systems such as the UK, it is wait-time–gated.

In a broken system where you can't get an appointment for six months, or can't afford to pay, the machine doesn't have to be perfect. It just has to be present and competent.

From wizard to pilot

Thinking bigger, we see that the algorithmic doctor is just the latest chapter in a very old story. For centuries, blue-collar workers have been the primary targets of technological disruption—from the textile weavers of the 19th century to the steel and auto workers of the 20th.

But in 2025, the crosshairs shifted upward. Teachers and coders found themselves on the front lines of AI displacement. Now, in 2026, the white-collar immunity has officially dissolved. Doctors, lawyers, and consultants are next. The ivory tower is not fireproof; it just burns last.

Culturally, we may see the social demotion of the physician. For millennia, the doctor was a **wizard**. Today's look at the murky gray shadows of an X-ray or the squiggly lines of an EKG and divine the truth. Magic. We trust them because we can't see what they see.

Now, the patient can see a "probability score" on their phone before the doctor. The doctor is shifting from wizard to **pilot**. We trust pilots, but we don't revere them. We just expect them to follow the checklist, trust the instruments, and land the plane without killing us.

We are entering an era of asymmetrical care. The patient, armed with AI, often knows more about their specific condition than the generalist they are paying to treat it. The doctor's role is shifting from "detective" to "contextualizer."

The interplay of truth and trust, from veneration to verification

Here we see the friction between **truth** and **trust** in its rawest form. AI provides a "truth" (a probability score, a diagnosis) that is around as good as a human one. But we lack the "trust" infrastructure to act on it.

We still require the human doctor to act upon the machine's truth, not because they are smarter, but because they are legally and socially accountable. We trust the person, even when the math says we should trust the machine. The next decade of medicine will be the slow**, painful transfer of that trust from the coat to the code**.

We are moving from institutional trust ("I trust you because you went to Harvard Med") to verifiable trust ("I trust you because your diagnosis matches the AI's probability score").

This feels like a loss of status for the profession, but for the patient, it is a massive gain in security. We are no longer relying on the "clinical judgment" of a single fallible human; we are relying on a consensus of millions of data points, checked by a human.

Thinking bigger: The economic collapse of the clinic

Will the economic model of the healthcare system survive the triumvirate? Right now, doctors are the "scrip gate"—the toll booth we must pass to get the medicine we need. But within five years, will that gate hold?

As home diagnostics (blood, saliva, biome) merge with diagnostic AI, the monopoly on prescription power will face intense pressure. We may see a bifurcation: "commodity care" (prescriptions for UTIs, rashes, statins) handled by AI with remote sign-off, and "complex care" reserved for the human expert.

The twelve-minute visit may be obsolete.

Thinking better: The trust triumvirate

This signals what may be a final collapse of medical paternalism; the third chair operating model is shifting from 'Doctor Knows Best' to 'Data Knows Best.' This turns the patient from a passive recipient of care into an active project manager of their own biology.

This system will run on trust. Doctors will no longer get away with being opaque about their decision-making criteria. They may have to be more open about uncertainty in diagnosis and prescription (how often today does a doctor say, "this (say) prescription, has a 70% success rate.") And trust in LLM's cannot be blind or uninformed – they make mistakes, and the biggest mistake we can make (as patients) is treating them as if they do not.

For human patients, this requires substantial new knowledge and skills, learning to interrogate the AI, to question it, to verify what it says, not just obey it.

But for all the upheaval this will cause during the next five years, I speculate that the standard of care will become much higher, as will patient literacy and self-advocacy.

Further reading

Topol, Eric. *Deep Medicine: How Artificial Intelligence Can Make Healthcare Human Again* (2019).

- *Why read it?* The seminal text on the "Centaur" model. Topol argues that AI won't replace doctors, but it will free them to focus on the one thing machines can't do: care.

"The AI Revolution in Medicine." *New England Journal of Medicine* (GPT-4 Special Report, 2024).

■ *Why read it?* A rigorous look at the "Third Chair" in practice. It details exactly where LLMs excel (diagnostics, paperwork) and where they fail (judgment), providing the clinical roadmap for the next five years.

"Overcoming Algorithm Aversion." *Harvard Business Review* (2025).

■ *Why read it?* Explains the psychology behind why we forgive a human doctor for killing a patient but lose our minds when an algorithm makes a minor error. Essential for understanding the "Trust Paradox."

"The Future of the Medical Profession." *The Lancet* (Digital Health Series)

■ *Why read it?* A systemic look at the "Scrip Gate," how the economics of the medical guild will crack under the pressure of democratized intelligence.

My Molecules, My Body

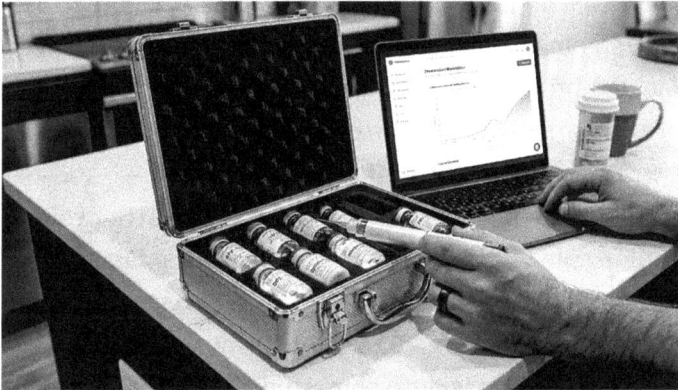

FIGURE 3.1: We've moved from a culture of fixing disease, to wellness, and now to optimization.

Peptides, self-doctoring, and the bodily autonomy wars

It happened on a couch in Costa Rica, the jungle outside, and the *White Lotus* rerun inside. Suddenly, my best buddy Dan lifted his shirt, pulled out an insulin syringe, and injected himself. Dan is 36, and non-diabetic, what was he up to?

Dan wasn't sick, he was optimizing. In fact, while injecting, he was also optimizing with red-light mask. He hasn't seen a seed oil, dairy, or sugar in a decade.

"Bro, what are you injecting?"

"HGH, growth hormone."

In fact, pure HGH is illegal and carries significant risks. Dan was injecting ipamorelin, a GH secretagogue peptide that stimulates HGH and Insulin-like Growth Factor (IGF) release. Its advertised benefits include increased muscle mass, faster exercise recovery, improved sleep, better skin and bone health, enhanced mood, and fat loss.

That moment was the canary in my coal mine where I witnessed the death of the passive patient and the birth of self-doctoring – the body as a **health project.** I spent five years of my early career doing lab work on peptides. To me, tinkering with the endocrine system was serious business. To Dan, it was just Tuesday.

Perhaps Dan is onto something. Certainly, the benefits advertised below made me want to borrow Dan's syringe.

The HGH evidence – benefits and risks

Dan was on the "hard stuff" of the biohacking world that includes peptides such as Body Protective Compound (BPC -157,) and ipamorelin, but also other bio-active molecules such as TRT (Testosterone Replacement Therapy), rapamycin, nicotinamide adenine dinucleotide (NAD)+, and ketamine.

For ipamorelin, there is reasonable, though mostly non-RCT (randomly controlled trial, the clinical gold standard) evidence for increasing GH/IGF-1 levels, improving sleep quality, supporting post-exercise recovery, and aiding modest fat loss through enhanced lipolysis.

So far so good.

Evidence is mixed for benefits on muscle gain, connective-tissue healing, and anti-inflammatory effects, with small human studies and animal data pointing in different directions. There is **no solid evidence** that ipamorelin increases lifespan, reverses aging, boosts cognition, meaningfully alters mood, or produces dramatic body-composition changes. The positives, then, are a mixed bag of somewhat probable, to remotely possible.

The risks, however, are very well defined: HGH has been studied extensively since discovered in 1956.

Chronically boosting GH and IGF-1 comes with well-established risks. Higher IGF-1 is linked to increased cancer risk and tumor growth, because it accelerates cell division and reduces apoptosis, giving any lurking malignancy a friendlier growth environment. It can also drive insulin resistance and higher blood sugar, nudging people toward prediabetes or diabetes, and cause fluid retention, joint pain, and carpal tunnel–type symptoms from soft-tissue overgrowth. With long-term, high exposure you also see concerns about cardiac remodeling (enlarged or stiffening heart) and subtle organ hypertrophy, which may not show up quickly but matter over years.

Then there's the big bucket of things we **don't really know**, especially in non-deficient people using peptides, TRT, or HGH for optimization. Many longevity researchers suspect that higher IGF-1 in mid- to late life shortens lifespan, even if it makes you feel and function better in the short term. But we don't yet have clean, long-term human data in biohacker-style dosing. It is also unclear how much GH/IGF-1 manipulation might wake up otherwise quiet cancers, how it affects brain aging, cognition, and mood over decades, and whether there is any safe "sweet spot" for nudging IGF-1 up without long-term trade-offs.

In short, short-term function and recovery may improve, but the long-term bill is uncertain and could be ugly. That has me worried about Dan.

From wellness to optimization

While indigenous cultures have always touted elixirs and potions, roots, herbs, rhino horn powders, orthodox medicine has stayed clear. In this century, wellness became a thing. (See the Wellness-industrial complex chapter, later.) This was the domain of yoga, mindfulness, fasting, juicing, and "detoxes." It was soft, feminine-coded, and largely harmless. It was a reaction to a medical system that felt rushed, indifferent, male, and mechanistic. It is also a seven trillion dollar industry projected to grow to ten trillion by the end of the decade. When folks ask what I think of the advice of a wellness guru, I usually respond, "I'd have to look at the specific research, but here is a guide. If they are selling **anything**, you should quadruple-check what they say."

Around 2023, the vibe shifted. We moved from wellness (feeling good) to optimization (performing better).

At the apex of this world sits Bryan Johnson, age 48, and his Blueprint longevity protocol. He's on the full longevity carnival ride: microdosing peptides, stacking metformin, rapamycin, and NAD boosters, blasting himself with red and near-infrared light, wearing continuous glucose monitors, doing cold plunges and sauna cycles, fasting, taking dozens of supplements, injecting exosomes and stem cells, getting full-body MRI scans, optimizing sleep with trackers and wearables, trying testosterone optimization, biohacking his microbiome, doing VO_2 max training, monitoring every biomarker imaginable, cycling nootropics, experimenting with mitochondrial enhancers, using AI diet plans, and posting the data like it's a religion.

This is more than health, this is biological engineering. And the demographic that follow Johnson isn't just bodybuilders or tech billionaires anymore. It is suburban dentists, accountants, and exhausted parents. They aren't going to their GP; they are going to Reddit, Telegram, and "research chemical" websites that ship vials labeled "NOT FOR HUMAN CONSUMPTION" directly to their doorsteps.

No metabolic free lunches

Biohackers treat optimization as a free metabolic lunch, a secure passage to a 120-year healthspan.

Some of these biohacking interventions seem more harmful and riskier, on balance, than beneficial. The "Barbie Peptide" (Melanotan II) is linked to cancer and the "Wolverine" shot (BPC-157) has no human safety trials. Experts urge caution. Some of Bryan Johnson's enhancements are demonstrably safe, others (for example metformin) carry substantial risks, but which are unsafe enough to ban?

There are added complications of risk timing and dose-dependency. Biohackers love **hormesis**, the idea that small doses of potentially harmful compounds are beneficial. That is, the dose-response curve is parabolic unlike traditional pharmaceuticals which have sigmoid curves, little effect at small dosages that increase until the effective dose is reached. (See Figure 3.2.)

The Dosage Paradox: Hormesis vs. Traditional Pharma

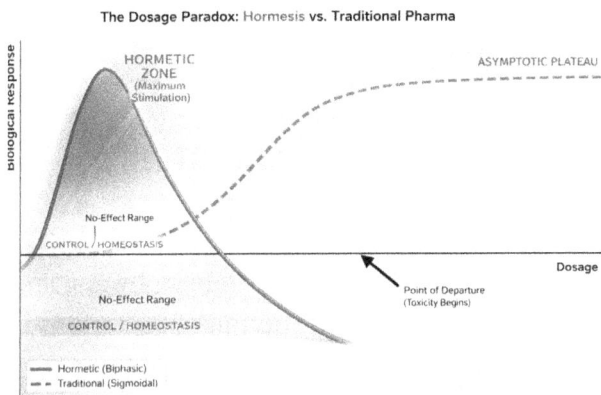

FIGURE 3.2: The hormesis dose-response curve compared with a standard drug

Timing also matters. If a molecule optimizes for someone in their thirties, but they will pay a severe price (cancer, premature death) in their 80s, should that be a choice they are allowed to make? And for many of the "hard stuff" compounds, we won't know for a generation what today's biohackers did to their bodies. It will be fifty more years to see how Bryan Johnson looks at 100.

Biohackers optimize for *today*; regulators worry about *tomorrow*.

The political philosophy of this is a "hard case," one unlikely to be resolved to anyone's satisfaction in 2026. The bodily autonomy crew, under the current cultural and regulatory milieu in the US, have won the argument. However, there is more to bodily autonomy than just biohacking. It affects the use of well-estab-lished treatments such as vaccination and statin use.

Trust in orthodox medicine, already on the run, is further compromised.

Libertarian biology and bodily autonomy

Where this trend hits political philosophy is complex. On the one hand, everyone, not just libertarians favor extensive individual rights – it is afterall, your body, and those are your molecules. The real battle is between individual rights and collective risk.

But under what conditions does the state have the right to protect us from ourselves? We (mostly) routinely accept some restrictions, speed limits, seatbelts, and fentanyl. But there are vast inconsistencies between policies and usage. The FDA bans BPC-157 while half of Silicon Valley injects it, stem cells are regulated as tightly than fentanyl, and psilocybin is Schedule I even as ketamine clinics pop up on every corner.

The central question of 2026 is: Who owns your biology?

We are seeing the rise of three distinct forms of medical autonomy that are dismantling the authority of the white coat.

Autonomy to OPT IN (The peak performer)

People are choosing to augment their baseline biology. The medical "Standard of Care" (SOC) says you treat a deficit; the "Optimizer" says you attack a plateau. The medical establishment views this as reckless; the user views it as essential maintenance for a high-performance life.

Autonomy to OPT OUT (The skeptic or sovereign individual)

The skepticism that began with vaccines and statins has calcified into a broader ideological stance: "My body is not a site for government policy." We are seeing a strange horseshoe theory in action where the left-leaning "Crunchy Mom" (who rejects GMOs) and the right-leaning "Tech Bro" arrive at the same conclusion: The system is poisoning us, and only we can fix it.

(And they have a point, the industrial food system is broken; ultra-processed, hyper-palatable foods are designed to part consumers from their dollars and not to nourish them. Where the types diverge is on regulation, Crunchy Mom sees too little regulation and unprotected kids, Tech Bro sees too much, inhibiting individual experimentation and innovation.)

Autonomy to OVERRIDE (The biohacker)

This is the most disruptive shift. People aren't just refusing the doctor's advice; they are also superseding it. They use AI to interpret their own labs. They order their own blood panels. They source their own compounds from China. The idea that you need a priest (Doctor) to speak to God (Biology) is dissolving. The Reformation is here, and Bryan Johnson is Martin Luther.

The economics of the gray zone

The risk here is not necessarily the molecules—peptides are elegant, naturally occurring signaling chains —it is the supply chain.

Because the FDA has cracked down on compounding pharmacies making these drugs (citing safety concerns, but effectively protecting big pharma IP), the market has gone underground. We have created a massive class divide in safety: The rich get prescriptions from boutique "longevity clinics" that charge $5,000 a month for clean, US-made peptides. The rest buy from the gray market accepting, consciously or not, the risk of contamination or inaccurate dosage.

My friend on the couch in Costa Rica is betting his liver on the quality control of a factory in Wuhan. He is crowdsourcing his safety data from anonymous anecdotes on Reddit.

The new trust architecture

This is the new **trust** architecture: We have stopped trusting institutions (the FDA, the AMA) and started trusting the network (the Discord server, the Huberman subreddit). It is distributed, fast, and democratic—but it is prone to dangerous cascades of misinformation.

This is a historic collapse in institutional trust and the rise of a new trust architecture. I read medical journals and *The New Scientist*; my biohacker, crypto-bro, and libertarian friends think those are corrupt and re-gressive. Their trusted sources are X, Reddit, Huber-man, and specialist biohacker forums.

To this trained scientist—albeit perhaps too much of a "credentialist," the plural of anecdote isn't data. I like big RCTs and databases full of clinical evidence (such as the Cochrane Collaboration.) This isn't a claim that evidence-based medicine is perfect; just that it is the best way we currently have of predicting whether a treatment will work or is safe.

To my biohacker buddies, an MD or PhD designa-tion is a cautionary signal; to me, those letters signal decades of scholarly enquiry, not (at least not initially) institutional capture or corruption.

When I ask, "Where did you get your information?" I feel the urge to throw up in my mouth when they cite a subreddit. They feel the same urge when I cite the *New England Journal of Medicine*.

Truth: the N-of-1 problem

The "Truth" for the optimizer is N=1. The optimizer doesn't care about randomized controlled trials; he cares that his tennis elbow disappeared after two weeks of BPC-157. This N=1 mindset feels rational because the data is personal: "I trust what my body tells me."

But individual experience is not population truth. The placebo effect is powerful, so powerful that even when people are told they are taking a placebo, there is an effect!

Beyond the placebo effect, the optimizer desperately wants to be right. Their identity is tied up with being ahead of the curve and being that little bit smarter than all those dumbass MDs and PhDs.

This creates an epistemic crisis. We are moving from Evidence-Based Medicine (population averages) to Experience-Based Medicine (individual variance). It feels like truth to the user, but to the scientist, it looks like dangerous hubris and self-deception. We have outsourced biomedical epistemology to the wisdom (and sometimes stupidity) of the crowd, applying sniper-grade decision-making to molecules sourced from group chats.

The 2026 horizon: the endocrine crash

By later this decade, I expect to see the first real consequences of the optimization boom. You cannot redline your endocrine system forever. A generation of men and women who have aggressively tinkered with their HPA (hypothalamic-pituitary-adrenal)—growth hormone, cortisol, testosterone, insulin, without understanding the long-arc feedback loops. The result will be down-regulation, receptor burnout, and hormonal instability. A new medical subfield will likely emerge, **recovery medicine**, whose sole purpose is cleaning up the biochemical wreckage of the self-engineered human.

But the genie isn't going back in the bottle.

Think bigger: the rise of the pharmacological self

The deeper questions are political. If I own my body, do I have the right to take risks with it that regulators call too risky? Libertarian Biology is a worldview in which bodily autonomy is absolute, and enhancement is a civil right. The optimizer doesn't see a peptide; he sees sovereignty. Whether society accepts or rejects this worldview will become one of the defining governance debates of the next decade. New technologies make that a safer choice, AI should power better "self-doctoring" decisions, but **libertarian mistrust of orthodox authority might also mean that AI's evidence-based guidance is easily dismissed**.

Think better: the mechanistic trap

But the intellectual trap of this movement is *mechanistic plausibility*. Biohackers mistake a working mechanism for a guaranteed outcome: "This peptide increases GH in vitro, so it will make me younger." Biology doesn't work like that. It's a complex adaptive system where pulling one thread (growth hormone) might unravel the entire sweater (cancer risk, insulin resistance, acromegaly).

Just because you know the mechanism doesn't mean you know the outcome. Mechanistic knowledge is not predictive knowledge. The optimizer thinks he is reading an engineering schematic; in reality, he is trying to predict how the climate system will respond based on temperature readings in Tulsa.

Further reading

The Science and Politics of Hormesis — Edward Calabrese (Toxicology and Applied Pharmacology)

- ■ *Why read it?* A foundational, rigorous review of dose-response curves, risks, and the misuse of hormesis in wellness and biohacking.

The Illusion of Evidence-Based Medicine — Jon Jureidini & Leemon McHenry

- ■ *Why read it?* A scathing, well-researched critique of how modern medicine arbitrates truth.

Drugs, Sex, and Biopolitics: The Pharmacological Turn in Selfhood — Nikolas Rose & Joelle Abi-Rached

- ■ *Why read it?* A scholarly but very readable look at how psychopharmacology, enhancement, and autonomy are reshaping the concept of the self.

CHAPTER I.4

GLP-1s and Identity-Editing

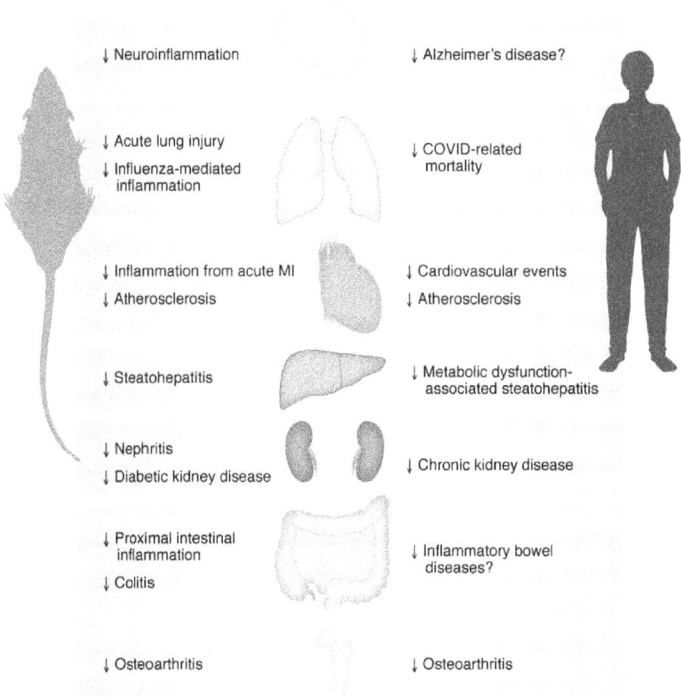

FIGURE 4.1: Anti-inflammatory actions of GLP-1 therapies
(Journal of Clinical Investigations)

The revolution we didn't see coming

"The GLP-1 drugs are the most important drug-class breakthrough in medical history," said acclaimed physician and researcher Eric Topol. Really? More important than antibiotics, vaccines, anesthesia, or insulin?

Sure, GLP-1 receptor agonists—originally developed for Type II diabetes—reliably produce 15–20% weight loss. Obesity, which affects roughly 40% of adults in many Western countries and drives a cascade of co-morbidities, may indeed be the most urgent public-health crisis we face.

But "in medical history"?

Still, Topol might be right.

The metabolic swiss army knife

Through physiological mechanisms we only dimly understand, these drugs appear to have wide-ranging effects far beyond the bathroom scale. Cardiovascular improvements appear long before much weight loss. One by one, trials reveal benefits unrelated to calorie deficit. Inflammation falls. The liver, kidneys, and even the brain show protective changes. Cognitive impairment slows in early Alzheimer's trials.

Cravings and addictive behaviors—smoking, alcohol, binge-eating, even compulsive impulses—often diminish as well. Sleep apnea improves. The "multipurpose agonist" framing is not hype; these drugs operate across a gut–brain–immune axis that scientists had barely mapped ten years ago.

But here's the part we're only beginning to grasp: they're not just reshaping bodies.

We are discovering that they rewire the mind, which reveals a fascinating and unanticipated mind-body connection. The drugs seem also to be **identity-editing molecules**—compounds that quietly reshape appetite, reward, self-concept, and the emotional scaffolding people use to navigate their daily lives.

The identity connection

The biggest impact of GLP-1s may not be the weight people lose, but the self-concepts they shed.

Via their effect on metabolism, patients lose on average around 15–20% of their body weight in a year. For those, like your author, who have been trying to lose the same thirty pounds for thirty years, the effect is dramatic.

However, the less-studied psychological effects may be as profound as the metabolic ones. When you subdue food cravings, you don't just flatten appetite; you flatten *all* appetitive impulses. Early studies and clinical anecdotes report declines in alcohol intake, smoking, binge-eating, gambling, pornography use, impulse shopping, and compulsive scrolling.

These results are preliminary, but they track precisely with what GLP-1 receptors do in the brain: modulate dopamine-linked reward valuation. We are not just medicating metabolism; **we are** also **editing the**

body's reward architecture. And when you rewire the reward architecture? Behaviors change.

It is the quiet silencing of craving pathways and hedonic loops that reshape emotional identity. Some experience this as relief, others as disorientation. For a subset, food was not just fuel; it was coping, ritual, or self-soothing. When that evaporates overnight, you don't just lose hunger—you lose part of who you were. The default coping mechanism of modern times—comfort eating—has been chemically severed.

And the new you may behave very differently.

Identity drives behavior; behavior drives identity

It is extremely difficult to change behavior. Studies on lifestyle adherence are grim; even after myocardial infarction, long-term adherence to diet and exercise changes hovers near 20-30%, dropping significantly over time. Since heart attacks happen at an advanced age, habits and reward pathways are "dug in." Social relationship and culture cement this: try quitting smoking in a family of smokers or switching to kale in a family that orders from Domino's. Behavioral science teaches us that sticky behaviors are resistant to conventional influencing, persuasion or education, but even to sharp emotional shocks, such as an MI.

GLP1s seem to work around that stickiness through their effect on reward pathways and "set points." We've known for years that weight has a biological set point—a defended equilibrium where hunger, satiety, metabolism, and brain chemistry all conspire to keep the body roughly the same size. Now it seems that identity has a set point, too. People carry an internal representation of who they are: how they eat, how they cope, what they desire, whom they desire, what they wear, and how they behave socially.

GLP-1s seem to erode both set points simultaneously. The body changes faster than the mind can update. The result is a peculiar form of identity lag: "I feel like myself, but not in my own body. I don't recognize who I am in the mirror."

Patients report they stop hiding in oversized clothes. They no longer build their day around dopamine hits from food. They abandon rituals—the late-night snack, the comfort dessert, or the bored fridge graze. Exercise was awkward; gyms were places where skinny people in Lululemon went.

Now patients may derive enjoyment. Hobbies such as hiking, dancing, and biking are pleasurable and possible when they once were not. Patients may have avoided dating; now they may not.

And while identity (one's self concept) may impede behavioral change because of its stickiness, when it starts to shift, behaviors follow, and altered behaviors shift identity – one may begin to identify a "as a gym rat" when one behaves as a gym rat does.

And when individual identities shift at the scale of 50 million people, it ceases to be psychology and becomes macroeconomics.

Thinking bigger: behavior affects society and economics

The food industry helps create and then exploits the obesity epidemic, hence, the "supersize me" culture. Foods can be designed, both in terms of ingredients and packaging, to encourage bingeing. But GLP-1s do more than shrink appetites; they expose a biological **truth** we have long ignored. For decades, we treated obesity as a failure of character—a deficit of willpower. The efficacy of these drugs proves it is partly a deficit of biology.

But, if tens of millions of people alter their reward circuitry, the food, alcohol, wellness, and healthcare industries must rewrite how they understand demand, risk, and behavior.

Obesity has shaped (pun intended) entire industries and identities: fashion, food, fitness, cosmetics, alcohol, retail, even aviation fuel consumption. A population-level appetite shift remaps all of these. Morgan Stanley estimates calorie consumption among GLP-1 users falls by 20–30%. Airlines save millions in fuel if the average passenger weight drops by ten pounds. The snack food industry is quietly panicking.

In wellness culture, the status hierarchy is already shifting: "disciplined" bodies versus "drug-assisted" ones; moralizing around "natural" weight loss versus "pharmaceutical" transformation. To the body purist, the injection is not medicine; it is **stolen valor**. Expect new forms of stigma, aspiration, and backlash, because identity changes ripple socially.

Layer AI onto this and you get something even more interesting. With continuous glucose monitors, wearables, AI-triage tools, and metabolic risk models, GLP-1 therapy becomes a platform for precision metabolic medicine. AI can predict who benefits most, who relapses, who develops side effects, and how to titrate safely.

When GLP-1s meet ambient intelligence, prevention shifts from advice to orchestration. This is still emerging, but it is the clearest path toward population-level reversal of metabolic disease in decades.

The frictions of 2026: economics vs. efficiency

By 2026, the GLP-1 landscape will shift from a handful of weekly jabs to a full ecosystem: daily pills, "Godzilla" triple-agonists like retatrutide, and new combinations designed to solve the "sarcopenia" problem—sparing essential muscle mass while stripping fat.

However, this medical miracle faces a market failure. **While the drugs work, the business model lags.** Insurers are stalling, trapped in short-termism. Why pay for a drug today when the savings (a prevented heart attack) won't materialize for ten years, likely when the patient is on a different insurance plan? This is the "wrong pocket" problem. The math is clear for society—treating obesity is cheaper than treating its complications—but it is messy for the payer.

Despite these economic frictions, the biological signal is impossible to ignore: GLP-1s are emerging as our first viable *geroprotectors* (anti-aging drugs). Recent research published in *Nature* highlights their mechanism: they do not just lower blood sugar; they systematically dampen "inflammaging"—the chronic, low-grade inflammation that drives frailty, Alzheimer's, and cardiovascular decay. By quieting the immune system's overreaction to modern life, **these molecules may be buying us not just thinner years, but *more* years**. We are inadvertently running the largest longevity clinical trial in human history, and the early results suggest we are slowing the biological clock.

This economic friction highlights a deeper tension: **Trust.** Patients must trust a pharmaceutical industry to maintain their new baseline for life; insurers must trust that preventative care yields ROI; and society must rebuild trust with a food system that has poisoned the well.

Thinking better: the band-aid or the cure?

GLP-1s are extraordinary molecules, but they sit on top of an obesogenic world: a food system built for hyper-palatable surplus and a lifestyle hostile to movement. In that sense, they are a band-aid on a deeper structural wound. They may even entrench a broken ecosystem by treating its downstream symptoms rather than its upstream causes.

Ultimately, the revolution is not just about size; it is about self. GLP-1s are identity interventions masquerading as metabolic ones. The challenge for the coming years is whether our institutions catch up to what the science already makes clear.

If your body changes faster than your mind, you need **wisdom, not just prescriptions**. You need new coping strategies, new self-stories, and a new form of health literacy to navigate a life where the "you" in the mirror is a stranger. We have found the chemical switch to turn off the noise of craving; now we must decide who we want to be in the quiet that follows.

GLP-1s are not a fad. They're not even primarily weight-loss drugs. They are identity interventions masquerading as metabolic ones—and identity changes at scale change society.

The challenge for 2026 is whether our institutions catch up to what the science, economics, and lived experience already make clear.

Further reading

Drucker, D. J. (2024). "GLP-1-based therapies: success, challenges, and future outcomes." Nature Metabolism.

- Why read it: This is the definitive "state of the union" from the scientist whose foundational research made Ozempic possible. It cuts through the hype to explain exactly how these molecules re-wire our metabolic operating system—and crucially, outlines the known unknowns that still keep scientists awake at night.

Hari, J. (2024). "Magic Pill: The Extraordinary Benefits and Disturbing Risks of the New Weight-Loss Drugs."

- Why read it: The necessary cultural counterweight. While scientists focus on the molecule, Hari focuses on the meaning. He explores the profound psychological and societal shockwaves of "solving" obesity with a weekly injection, questioning whether we are liberating ourselves from food noise or merely outsourcing our self-regulation to Big Pharma.

Lincoff, A. M., et al. (2023). "Semaglutide and Cardiovascular Outcomes in Obesity without Diabetes (SELECT Trial)." The New England Journal of Medicine.

- Why read it: The study that changed everything. Before SELECT, Wegovy was a "lifestyle drug." After SELECT proved a 20% reduction in heart attacks and strokes—it became "healthcare." This is the data that forced insurance companies to pay attention and transformed GLP-1s from a cosmetic luxury into a systemic medical necessity.

The Wellness-Industrial Complex

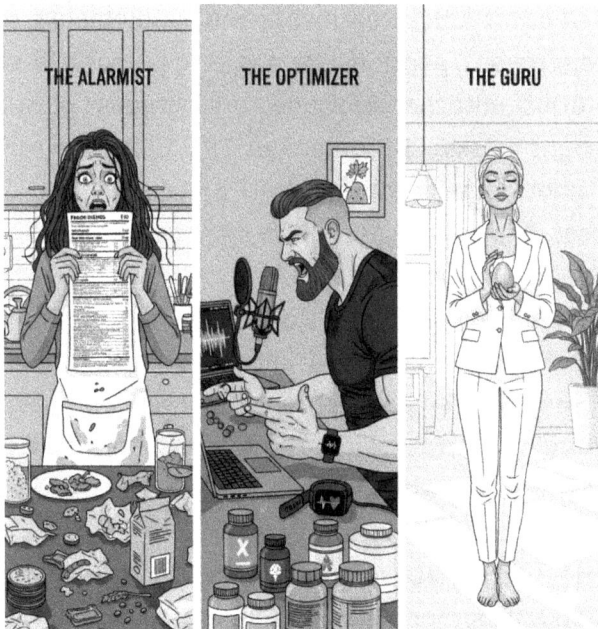

FIGURE 5.1: The archetypes of wellness-industrial influencers (any resemblance to known persons is ~~intentional~~ purely accidental)

Bodily freedom or public health menace?

In the 2000s, the supplement ephedra began killing people. People taking the supplement developed toxic cardiomyopathy, and it was eventually banned. The end of unregulated supplements, you might think? Nope.

The wellness economy, of which supplements are a part, has swollen into a $5.6 trillion parallel medical universe. Walk into any Walgreens and you'll face 500+ supplements promising energy, immunity, longevity, detoxification, better sleep, better mood, or better skin.

Add to that a more modern assortment of unregulated or off-label treatments and supplements, such as adaptogens, peptides, saunas, cold plunges, IV-vitamin drips, mitochondrial boosters, "greens" powders, red-light masks, CBD gummies, TRT, GLP-1 microdosing, nootropic chocolates, NAD precursors, and CGM devices, and you see one of the main healthy behaviors of the modern "worried well."

There is no good medical evidence for any of this (see below for what "good" means.) On the *Think Bigger, Think Better* podcast, anti-quackery campaigner Dr. Stephen Barrett said, "The evidence for **most** supplements, for **most** people is that all they give you is expensive pee."

Most of the above are harmless as well as effectless, so why bother? People can spend their money how they please. However, as we will see, there are systemic downsides, including the corruption of trust and truth.

Double standards, or freedom to augment?

For a drug or procedure to pass regulatory approval, generally a controlled trial (RCT) must be conducted, one group receiving the treatment, and the other a placebo or the current standard of care. (There are much more complex versions.)

Over long-time-scales and large sample sizes, both efficacy and an acceptable safety profile must be demonstrated. This is far from perfect because big pharma knows how to game the system, but it is the best method known for deciding what products can be marketed and sold as medicine.

This is the first conflict. Approvals can be glacially slow. The process is conservative—many drugs fail, and treatments that might safely help some people do not make it through the hoops. Moreover, the process costs real money. To shepherd a drug through Phase III trials may cost billions, designer peptides and treatments don't have a large enough TAM (total addressable market.)

Most substances in the wellness economy—from nootropics to peptides to proprietary supplement blends—bypass this architecture entirely. They do not have to go through any of that.

That places the wellness industry in an economic sweet spot, a huge market, with little accountability (for results or for risks). You would be hard to find another product in the world that is like this.

Pharma is guilty until proven innocent; wellness is innocent until proven guilty

This leaves evidence evaluation with the consumer who may or may not have taken 10th-grade chemistry. The wellness universe runs its $7 trillion economy on hopium, cognitive biases, and charisma-coated greed. We look at them—gorgeous, jacked, radiating vitality— and our primitive brain whispers, *"All this stuff must work, right?"*

In one worldview, these influencers are rene- gades—agile heroes steps ahead of a slow, ossified medical system. In the contrary view, they are preda- tors and the rest of us are prey.

The influencer ecosystem is split on how they use science. At the bottom are the aesthetic influencers who don't pretend to be science-literate; they simply say, "Look at me! I am beautiful/rich/fit—buy this tea."

But at the top end, the game is different. These are the influencers who wrap their merch in a coat of science. (And make no mistake: at this level, everyone is selling something—whether it is a proprietary sup- plement line, an affiliate code for greens powder, or a subscription to "exclusive" protocols.)

This is where the danger lies. People listen to the biochemistry word salad and even though they have no idea what NAD+ does, or what oxidative phosphoryla- tion is, it sounds sciency so they buy.

The biochemical slaughterhouse

Ask yourself, why do diabetics have to inject insulin (a peptide made of 51 amino acids) rather than just swallow a pill? If the supplement is a protein or peptide (like collagen, glutathione, or BPC-157), swallowing it is useless. Your body treats it like a steak—it dices it up into tiny molecular components. To use many compounds as a medicine, you have to inject them.

The stomach is a **biochemical slaughterhouse**. It is designed to be hostile. With a pH of 1.5–2.0 and a bath of aggressive enzymes like pepsin, its evolutionary mandate is to dismantle macromolecules—proteins, peptides, exotic herbal extracts, and $80 collagen powders—into their generic, constituent parts.

Nothing complex survives intact.

- **The routing error:** You cannot "target" nutrition. When you eat collagen, your body breaks it down into generic amino acids. The body then decides where those amino acids go based on survival needs, not your vanity. It might use them to repair a gut lining or build a heart valve, not to smooth your forehead.
- **The gauntlet:** Even if a molecule survives the acid, it faces the liver's **first-pass metabolism** and the kidneys' ruthless filtration. Megadosed Vitamin C? You will simply excrete expensive pee within hours. Oral glutathione? Usually destroyed before it hits the bloodstream.

And don't get me started on *topical* collagen. Collagen molecules are physically too large to penetrate the epidermis. They sit on top and moisturize; they do not rebuild structure. Synthesis is an anabolic internal process, not a topical paint job.

Even if a molecule works in a petri dish, and even if it works in a mouse, it still faces the ultimate barrier: your own anatomy.

This is the bioavailability fallacy, the widespread misunderstanding of what happens when we swallow "antioxidant-rich" foods or delicate supplements. We imagine these molecules traveling intact to our cells to scrub away rust. We confuse what is *in the pill* with what survives to end up *in the tissue*.

This central confusion fuels the wellness industry: the belief that the stomach is a passive entry gate—a mailbox where you deposit a "skin molecule" and it gets delivered to your skin.

Finally, we must respect the body's obsession with **homeostasis**. Your body is not a sandbox you can play in; it is an equilibrium machine operating within deadly narrow tolerances.

- A shift of just 0.5 mEq/L in potassium can stop your heart.
- A sodium change of 5–10 mEq/L can trigger seizures.

The body fights rapid change because rapid change usually means death. The notion that a scoop of "metabolic optimization powder" is allowed to meaningfully alter these parameters is physiologically incoherent. If it worked the way influencers claim, it would likely kill you.

While the bio-availability fallacy powers influencer sales, they have more prestidigitation at their disposal.

If you *must* take a pill, look for liposomal delivery (encasing the molecule in a fat bubble to sneak it past the acid) or enteric coating (a shell that doesn't melt until it hits the alkaline environment of the intestines).

The evidence gap: mice are not men (or women)

Since most consumers don't know biochemistry or physiology, wrapping a product in science works. Here are the convincing-sounding science cheats they use:

The first cheat is the **naturalistic fallacy**, an ancient heuristic that has metastasized into modern marketing. It operates on the simple, flawed logic that "natural" equals virtuous and "synthetic" equals toxic. We instinctively recoil from "chemicals" like Ozempic while embracing "supplements" derived from obscure roots, conveniently forgetting that nature is the world's most prolific manufacturer of poisons—cyanide, arsenic, and botulinum are all 100% natural. Conversely, the "unnatural" inventions of eyeglasses, antibiotics, and sewage treatment are the only reason many of us are alive to debate this.

The second distortion is the **placebo-by-price bias**, often called the "Chivas Regal Effect." In the absence of biochemical literacy, we use price as a proxy for potency. A $500 vitamin IV drip feels efficacious not because of the vitamins, but because of the $500 price tag. We are buying the feeling of efficacy. The brain releases endogenous opioids in anticipation of a reward, and the magnitude of that release often scales with the magnitude of the investment. We don't just pay for the treatment; we pay for the belief that it works.

(Personal note: my prospective in-laws in 2000 worked hard for their money in union jobs. Visiting their Ohio home, I saw them mixing up green goo in a morning smoothie. These were "liquid vitamins" and cost $500 a month - $1000 in today's money, and about as much as their mortgage. I suggested that a) they probably didn't need vitamins at all as healthy adults, and b) that the pills at CVS, while less sexy, cost $11, and c) a molecule was a molecule whether you consumed it in liquid form or capsule. This input was not well-received, a "doctor" – probably an MLM scammer – had "prescribed" them – for which ailments I never found out. But the serious point is that these folks with only high school science had been science-conned into spending their house payment on treatments they didn't need.)

The third distortion is **survivor bias**, the engine of the influencer economy. We look at the shredded podcaster hawking bone marrow supplements and assume the causal link: the supplements made him shredded. In truth, we are seeing the genetic lottery winner who would likely be ripped eating sawdust. We fail to see the invisible graveyard of 10,000 others who took the same stack but stayed soft. We mistake the survivor for the proof, confusing genetic inputs for pharmaceutical outputs.

The fourth distortion is the **mechanistic fallacy**, often disguised as "cutting-edge science." Mechanistic plausibility ("this molecule activates AMPK in vitro") is presented as clinical effectiveness ("you will live longer"). This is the error of confusing biological plausibility with clinical reality.

Influencers love to cite studies showing that a compound "optimizes mitochondrial pathways" or "activates longevity genes" in a petri dish or a lab mouse. They sell the mechanism (how it might work) as proof of the outcome (that it really works). But human biology is not a linear machine; it is a chaotic, adaptive system. A compound that extends life in a worm may do nothing—or cause cancer—in a primate. Influencers would like you to believe that what happens in a sterile, assuming that what happens in a sterile dish translates to the messy reality of the human body.

The quiet revolution: an epistemic restructuring

This isn't just a health fad; it is a fundamental shift in how society determines what is "true." We have undergone a migration:

- **From institutional trust to aesthetic authority:** We moved from trusting clinicians—guided by evidence, training, and standards—to trusting influencers fueled by charisma, relatability, and "the looks."

- **Lowering standards, raising personalization:** Each step of this migration lowers the requirement for evidence while increasing the appeal of "bespoke" or "personalized" marketing.

- **The swap of competence for confidence:** We have traded the quiet, nuanced accuracy of the expert for the loud, unwavering certainty of the amateur.

- **The circulation of truth:** This restructuring makes it increasingly difficult for objective truth to circulate, as it is constantly drowned out by high-production-value misinformation.

The optimization traffic light: a critical taxonomy

Navigating the wellness landscape requires an epistemic filter and some willingness to dig deeper into the science than most have time for. Humans, however, reach for the credit card before the medical journal. There is no excuse for this today. Every LLM will summarize the science, the benefits, and the risks based on the latest research in under a minute. You can still ignore it.

But be warned, LLMs are trained on internet science. One LLM "pro-tip" is to tell it what to consider and ignore. For example, Claude doesn't know me and unlike the LLMs I use more often, it doesn't know what I expect. So when I did a quick "double-check" on bone marrow supplements (useless) it fed me information from WebMD and Healthline. Moreover, it gave me their findings "raw" – that is, uncritically, when they were talking nonsense. (See Figure 5.2 for me giving it a slap on the wrist.) If you like Huberman, who millions do, make sure you use an LLM and ask "what evidence from medical journals is there to support his claim?" (It depends what he is talking about, when he sticks to his lane, he is on point – however, he isn't a biochemist, physiologist, pharmacologist, or nutritionist, and he sells all manner of sus products.) For a Huberman alternative that sticks to the evidence, try the **Maintenance Phase podcast.**

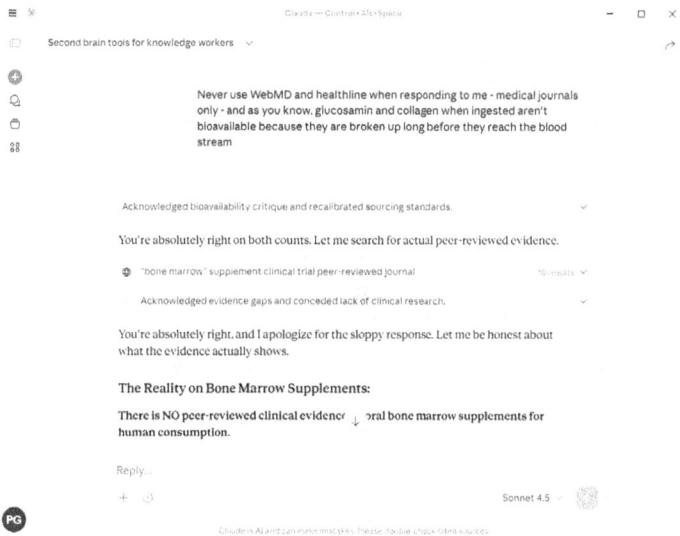

FIGURE 5.2: If you don't tell LLMs what your standards for knowledge are, you may get internet bullshit.

The following table (Figure 5.3) is a research-based heuristic, a traffic light system designed to separate biological signal from marketing noise. It is based on current clinical consensus, but it serves as a guide rather than a universal prescription. While the influencer economy treats every new compound as a miracle, the clinical reality is often a spectrum ranging from non-negotiable to total scam.

The most critical variable in this matrix is *context*. In biology, there are rarely universal "good" inputs, only appropriate ones. Vitamin D, for example, is a life-saving intervention for a deficient nursing home resident but metabolically useless for a replete twenty-year-old. Ashwagandha works as a tactical brake on acute stress, yet chronic use may lead to emotional flatness. Red light therapy shows promise for surface-level dermatology but cannot penetrate deep enough to "heal organs." The verdict often depends less on the molecule and more on the *milieu*—who is taking it, and why.

Finally, we must distinguish between *toxicity* and *futility*. The vast majority of red-light supplements, such as proprietary "Greens Powders," are safe enough; their crime is not poisoning you but rather generating expensive pee. Similarly, while influencers hawk oral collagen for glowing skin, your stomach acid ruthlessly dismantles it into generic amino acids long before it reaches your face. Those amino acids go where they are most needed in the body, not straight to the wrinkles on your face.

In the table below, a Red Light rarely warns of danger; it warns of the sophisticated transfer of wealth from your bank account to their shareholders.

The optimization traffic light: a critical taxonomy

PROTOCOL / SUPPLEMENT	INFLUENCER CLAIM	THE CLINICAL REALITY	EFFECTIVENESS	POTENTIAL HARM
Creatine	Muscle, cognition	Massive RCT evidence for strength; emerging data for brain health.	● SOLID	▮▯▯▯▯
Folate (B9)	Pregnancy health	Non-negotiable for fetal neural tube development. Real medicine.	● MANDATORY	▮▯▯▯▯
Vitamin D	Immunity, mood	Vital if deficient; useless or toxic if replete. Context is key.	◐ CONTEXTUAL	▮▮▯▯▯
Magnesium	Sleep, anxiety	Good evidence for sleep quality/RLS. One of the few effective minerals.	● LIKELY	▮▯▯▯▯
Sauna	Longevity, heart	Strong observational data (Finland). Likely mimics cardio exercise.	◐ LIKELY	▮▮▯▯▯
Cold Plunge	Dopamine, fat loss	Spikes dopamine/noradrenaline. Blunts muscle growth post-workout.	◐ MIXED	▮▮▯▯▯
Ashwagandha	Stress, T-levels	Lowers cortisol. Long-term safety unknown; risk of emotional numbing.	◐ TAKE BREAKS	▮▮▮▯▯
COM (Non-diabetic)	Metabolic control	No benefit for healthy people. Drives anxiety and disordered eating.	◐ ANXIETY	▮▮▮▯▯
Metformin (Healthy)	Anti-aging	Great for diabetics; in healthy people, it blunts exercise benefits.	○ BACKFIRES	▮▮▮▯▯
Turmeric	Inflammation	Poor bioavailability. Works in a petri dish, rarely reaches the blood.	○ BIOAVAILABILITY	▮▯▯▯▯
Red Light Therapy	Mitochondria	Promising for surface skin; cannot penetrate to deep organs.	◐ SKIN DEEP	▮▮▯▯▯
NMN / NAD+	Reverse aging	The 'Sinclair' effect. Impressive in mice; human trials failed to replicate.	○ HYPE	▮▮▯▯▯
Collagen (Oral)	Skin, joints	Digested into generic amino acids. The body routes them, not you.	○ HYPE	▮▯▯▯▯
Greens Powders	'Insurance'	Expensive 'dusting' of ingredients hidden behind proprietary blends.	○ HYPE	▮▯▯▯▯
IV Drips	Detox, hydration	Useless for healthy kidneys. Purely performative wellness.	○ HYPE	▮▮▯▯▯

©Paul Gibbons 2026 · INFORMATIONAL USE ONLY. NOT MEDICAL ADVICE.

FIGURE 5.3: A rough guide to the effectiveness and potential harm of some popular influencer therapies and products.

Your homework: don't trust me or the influencer. Trust the science

I could fill this page with citations that you won't read, and frankly, you shouldn't trust anyone, Huberman or me, without verification. In an era of "science-washing," influencers use the word *research* to mean "I found one obscure paper that supports my product."

If you want to opt out of the marketing matrix, you need independent auditors, that is, organizations that do not sell pills. Before you spend $100 on a bottle of hope, check these three databases:

1. **Examine.com:** The gold standard for nutrition. They analyze every study on a supplement and tell you if it works, does nothing, or is dangerous. They take no industry funding.
2. **The Cochrane Library:** The highest tier of Evidence-Based Medicine. If Cochrane says there is "insufficient evidence," it means the product is unproven, no matter what the podcast said.
3. **NCCIH (NIH):** The National Center for Complementary and Integrative Health. The US government's sober, boring, and highly accurate take on everything from acupuncture to zinc.

If it isn't validated by one of these three, you are not a bio-hacker; you are a customer.

Why the only cost isn't just expensive pee

The standard medical critique of wellness, that it is mostly harmless, just "expensive pee," misses the true scale of the damage. If the only cost were torching $50 on a bottle of multivitamins, we could shrug and move on. But the costs are not merely financial; they are also systemic. We are witnessing a massive transfer of authority.

When we normalize the idea that a podcaster's anecdote is equal to a randomized controlled trial, we are not just buying supplements; we are also outsourcing our epistemology. We are training a generation to trust charm, appearance, and word-salads over institutional research.

The danger is not the supplement itself, but the erosion of the cognitive baseline. When the next pandemic or public health crisis hits, millions will not look to the CDC for guidance. They will look to YouTube.

We are dismantling the infrastructure of public trust, brick by brick, in exchange for the feeling of control.

Wellness is not harmless fluff. It is a new epistemic regime shaping how humans understand their own biology. The central question of modern health is no longer "What is the cure?" but **"**Who has earned the right to tell us what is real?"

In this environment, **evidence literacy** becomes a civic skill, not just a medical one. The hierarchy of evidence—once guarded by universities and journals—must be rebuilt internally by every citizen. We have entered an era where truth is a consumer product, and **trust** is the most valuable currency of all.

The unstoppable machine: until another ephedra?

If you need proof that this economy is bulletproof, look at the ghost of ephedra. In the early 2000s, this stimulant killed people—causing cardiac hypertrophy, arrhythmias, and strokes in healthy users. When the ban finally came, experts predicted the unregulated wellness economy would implode under the weight of its own danger.

Instead, it grew faster. The industry simply pivoted, swapped molecules, and kept selling. This is the case study that proves the thesis: the supplement economy is not stoppable. It is protected by the 1994 DSHEA legislation that handcuffed the FDA, fueled by a **health freedom** narrative that appeals equally to the crunchiest liberal and the most ardent libertarian, and guarded by a lobbying apparatus that rivals big pharma.

Thinking bigger: could we, should we stop any of this?

The political reality is that the genie is out of the bottle, and the cork is long gone. Society cannot police a $5.6 trillion decentralized marketplace where truth is now a customized algorithmic feed. We cannot regulate our way out of this because the desire for these products is not medical, it is psychological.

We are left with a stark trajectory. We have seen the move from powders to **peptide culture**—a shift toward injectables that carries the risk of a massive, silent endocrine crash. We see the rise of AI-personalized stacks and algorithmic wellness coaches that reinforce our biases rather than challenging them.

The market will likely fracture into two distinct

tribes: "Aesthetic Wellness" (looking good at any cost) and "Evidence-Based Longevity" (actual risk reduction). The government is powerless to stop the former, so it falls to the individual to choose the latter.

Thinking better: we are buying connection and agency, not health

Why has this happened? Because orthodox medicine, for all its miracles, has become cold, bureaucratic, and reactive. Influencers build relationships with followers that provide **connection** – a stark contrast to the perceived distance of a doctor-patient relationship.

People are hungry for **agency**. In a world of chaotic variables, adhering to a strict morning protocol provides a secular liturgy, a way to quell anxiety and perform control. We buy these products not just to optimize our mitochondria, but also to soothe our minds. We are competing for more well than thou status in a society that conflates biological optimization with moral virtue.

Further reading:

Raphael, Rina. *The Gospel of Wellness: Gyms, Gurus, Goop, and the False Promise of Self-Care* (2022).

- ◼ *Why read it?* This is the definitive cultural autopsy of the $5.6 trillion beast. Raphael doesn't just mock the industry; she explains why it works—how the medical system's cold bureaucracy created a vacuum that influencers were happy to fill with connection and agency.

Offit, Paul A. *Do You Believe in Magic? The Sense and Nonsense of Alternative Medicine* (2013).

- *Why read it?* Dr. Offit is the bulldog of evidence-based medicine. This book contains the specific, horrifying history of the DSHEA legislation and the Ephedra crisis you mentioned. If you want the legal and medical "receipts" on how the supplement industry managed to deregulate itself into immortality, this is the source code.

Ehrenreich, Barbara. *Natural Causes: An Epidemic of Wellness, the Certainty of Dying, and Killing Ourselves to Live Longer* (2018).

- *Why read it?* Ehrenreich dismantles the "Control" narrative, arguing that our obsession with optimization is a secular religion designed to distract us from the reality of death. It attacks the "virtue signaling" of cellular health and provides the perfect counterweight to the "more well than thou" culture.

www.ingramcontent.com/pod-product-compliance
Lightning Source LLC
Chambersburg PA
CBHW060634210326
41520CB00010B/1597